OVERCOMING SICKNESS

God's Guidance
for Ultimate Health in Body,
Mind and Spirit

Michael Peters, M.D.

DEDICATION

To JESUS

His unconditional love has changed my life

CONTENTS

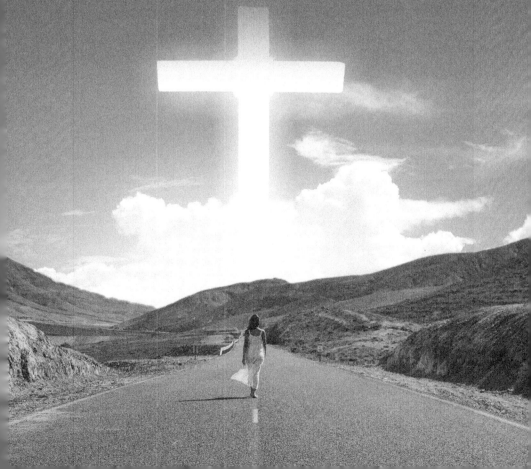

Chapter 1

THE JOURNEY BEGINS

s it possible to be free from sickness? The answer is a resounding yes! The purpose of this book is to help people struggling with all types of sickness or disease move into divine health. Having a healthy body, mind, and spirit is necessary to experience divine health. Not only is it possible to recover from your current illness, but it is possible to remain free of sickness.

Do your health problems feel like heavy weights you can no longer carry? Listen to Linda's story.

"I'm sorry; there is no cure for your type of cancer." Stunned by the doctor's words, Linda burst into tears. Years of poor health had finally culminated in this diagnosis. Linda had a long history of struggling with diabetes, which contributed to her anxiety and depression. The years of endless treatments, medications, and visits to the doctor had taken its toll. Weary and tired, Linda was losing hope. She wondered who was going to take care of her family. Simple work around the house was difficult because of fatigue and loss of energy. Linda had always loved getting together with friends and family, but now she had limited mobility. In the midst of this overwhelming diagnosis, Linda experienced a ray of hope. Linda learned about the principles laid out in this book, and she used these truths to move into divine health. Just like Linda, you can receive hope and healing in your life.

MY STORY

How does a doctor trained in the medical profession get involved in divine healing? My personal journey began when one of my sons received a diagnosis of depression. The symptoms had developed slowly. My wife, Mary Jo, and I were unaware of the serious nature of his illness. Even though our son received excellent medical care, we realized the medication and the treatment were not curing his problem, but were simply masking his symptoms.

The crisis began when we heard the words no parent ever wants to hear. "Your son has taken an overdose of medication, and it is life-threatening."

While racing to the hospital, my wife and I were fervently praying. In the emergency room, not knowing if our son would live or if he would have permanent health problems, I received a text from a friend. The friend simply texted me the words, "God said that your son will recover." Instantly, Mary Jo and I were filled with a peace that can only come from God. We just knew that our son would be okay. Our son remained in the hospital for three days, but he completely recovered and had no complications.

It was then that my wife and I fully realized that God created human beings with a body, mind, and spirit. For a person to walk in divine health, we now understood that the spirit and mind of a person had to be healthy along with the health of their physical body. With encouragement from my wife and me, our son pursued health in his spirit, mind and body. He overcame his depression and is still living free of all symptoms.

What Mary Jo and I discovered, we are now using to help others who are battling physical, mental, spiritual, and/or emotional illness. We have coached many people struggling with sickness into divine health. The same principles are effective for any type of disease or illness. We also understand you most likely have tried to get answers through other means and have not found the hope and healing you desire.

It is our joy to share our expertise and compassion to help you navigate your journey to divine health. We know God is a miracle-working God, and we believe you are His next miracle.

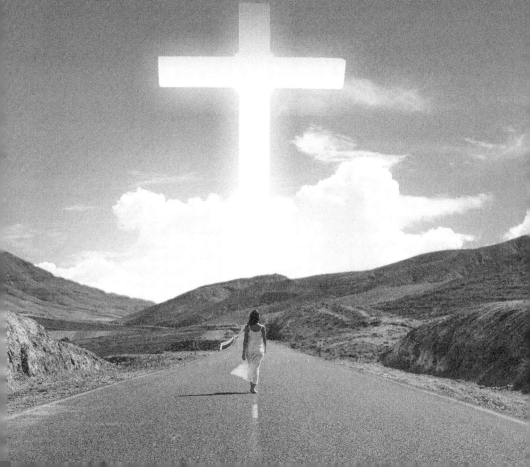

Chapter 2

KNOWING YOUR POSITION WILL CHANGE YOUR CONDITION

Y ou may be asking, "How do I begin?"

It starts by knowing your identity in Christ, and what He has already done for you. When we know our position, we can change our condition. Once we see all that Jesus has provided for us, we can simply receive it and make it part of our lives. Jesus has already given us the gift of healing. What a blessing and privilege! Many people are waiting upon God to bring healing to them, but really, He is waiting for us. God wants us to understand that we just have to accept the healing that He has already provided through Jesus.

When an individual becomes a believer in Jesus, they are immediately given power over sin, sickness, and the enemy. This does not mean they are perfect and never sin or get sick.

It simply means that we can overcome the sin and sickness in our lives through Jesus and His promises in the Bible.

Our mind needs to be transformed by the Word of God. We must change the way we think. If we think we will never get well or that God wants us to suffer with our illness, it becomes difficult to experience healing. God's will for you is healing and restoration. As our mind is renewed to this truth, our speech will follow, and this will lead to change in our actions or behavior.

One of the main reasons Christians fail to receive divine health is they think about their problems instead of God's promises. When Sara started focusing on God's promises, her life changed. Sara will tell you what happened in her own words.

"I have struggled with depression, anxiety, and heartburn for many years. I have seen multiple doctors, counselors, and therapists, but none of them could give me the healing I desperately wanted. When I met Dr. Michael Peters, he was different. He encouraged me to trust God and showed me how to change my destructive ways of thinking. He and his wife, Mary Jo, were very kind and loving to me. The process took some time, but Michael and Mary Jo never gave up on me and prayed faithfully for me. Through his compassionate coaching, I was able to know and experience the love of Jesus in my life. I am now living a life of hope and peace, completely healed of all my depression, anxiety, and heartburn. I am grateful to Jesus for healing me."

When an individual has thoughts of fear, doubt, anxiety, hopelessness, or unbelief, they are focusing on their negative circumstances. Instead, their attention should be on what God says in the Bible. The Scriptures are full of verses on healing, hope, peace, and building faith.

I have a free gift for you on my website: www.divinehealingcoach.com. This gift includes some powerful scriptures that you can use to pray as you begin your journey to divine health.

When you start on this journey into divine health, some people will criticize you and will not understand. Again, you must put your trust in God's promises and not listen to negative comments from other people. I would encourage you to find two or three healing verses in the Bible that are specific to the type of healing you are seeking. Then, it is important to speak these healing verses out loud every day. This only takes a few minutes a day, but it is powerful. It is also important to write down the specific areas of healing that you desire in your life. This will increase your hope and faith in God's healing.

Knowing the difference between hope and faith will guide you to receive healing. Hope simply means expectation. Hope causes you to see the promises of God in His Word as your future destination. First, find healing verses in the Bible that are specific to your life situation. Then place your hope in these scripture verses. We have a hope in God's promises in the Bible because we know they are true. Having hope leads to faith.

"Faith is the substance of things hoped for, the evidence of things not seen" (Heb 11:1 KJV). Faith is the confident assurance that God will do what He says He will do. In order to have faith in the present, you must have hope for the future. Faith becomes active when hope has revealed a destination from a promise in the Word of God. The following is an example of how hope and faith work together. An individual was recently diagnosed with lung cancer. This person chooses Psalm 103:3, which speaks about the Lord healing all your diseases. This verse is where they place their hope, because that is their final destination of healing. Faith is simply believing this Bible promise while they are going through the healing process. Faith enables the person to overcome their sickness because they are choosing to believe the healing promise from God instead of the doctor's report. Trusting in someone other than the Lord will lead to disappointment. Having faith in God and His promises will never disappoint you.

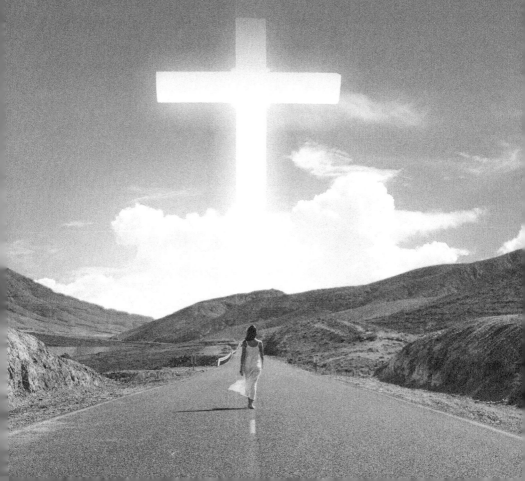

Chapter 3

HEALING IS FOR TODAY

Have you tried to find answers for your health with no success? I have good news for you. It is God's will for you to be healed. The Old and New Testament contain many powerful healing verses. Jesus is the same yesterday, today, and forever. We know Jesus healed many people on earth 2000 years ago, and Jesus has also used His disciples to release healing to multitudes of people. Jesus is still healing today because He desires to show His love and compassion to hurting people.

A woman named M. C. was diagnosed with a malignant brain tumor in June, 2022. The doctor said that even with surgery and treatment, she would only have a few months to live. She was fearful and felt hopeless because the medical prognosis was so devastating. She had surgery at Mayo

Clinic and had a complication of bleeding in her brain afterwards. A few months later, she attended one of our healing services. The following are her words telling what happened.

"I attended a healing service led by Dr. Michael Peters in September 2022. During the service, Michael called me out and asked me to come forward. Michael told me that Jesus was healing me of my brain cancer, and then he and his wife prayed for me. Two weeks later, I had a follow up appointment at Mayo Clinic. I received an amazing report!! The doctors told me I could go back to work, because they could not find any evidence of the brain tumor, and the brain bleed had vanished. I am extremely grateful that Jesus gave me my life back."

What Jesus did for M. C., He also wants to do for you. No matter what sickness or disease you are struggling with, God's plan for you is divine health.

It is clear from the Bible that Jesus suffered, died on the cross, and rose from the dead. After the resurrection, Jesus received all authority in heaven and on earth. Jesus then gave all His followers that same authority over sickness, disease, and the devil. Jesus paid the price on the cross to forgive our sins and heal our bodies. We do not have to suffer with our illnesses because Jesus already paid the price for our healing.

A connection exists between sin and sickness. This does not mean that if you sin once or unknowingly that you will get sick. It means that if you willingly continue to commit sin, sickness can affect your life. Not all disease is caused by sin, but chronic sin can open the door to physical illness. When we acknowledge our sins and confess them to Jesus, He will forgive our sins and bring healing to our spirit, mind, and body.

One reason people do not receive their healing is because they have heard incorrect teaching or information. This can cause doubt or unbelief. The Bible reveals the truth about healing. When people hear the truth and believe it, they will experience divine health.

There are three steps in this healing process. First, realize that it is God's will for you to be healed. Second, find healing scriptures in the Bible and believe them. Third, speak those promises of healing out loud daily. Speaking the promises of God out loud for even a few minutes a day is powerful.

My wife and I used these same principles when one of our sons was born with an eye ailment. He would wake up every morning with his eye completely stuck shut. We tried different medications and treatments for one year, but nothing worked. The eye doctor told us that our son would need surgery to correct this problem. As my wife and I prayed, we did not feel any peace about our son having the surgery. We felt God had another plan, so we decided not to have the surgery. Shortly after our decision, we met a man who prayed for us. He told us that God was going to heal our son soon. One week after that man prayed for us, our son woke up, and his eye was completely normal for the first time since he was born. Our son had no more problems with his eye, and that was many years ago.

As a physician who practiced medicine for 30 years, I know God uses doctors and nurses to bring healing to people. I also know that God releases healing through natural and supernatural methods. God is not limited to any one area. The next chapter focuses on natural ways God heals.

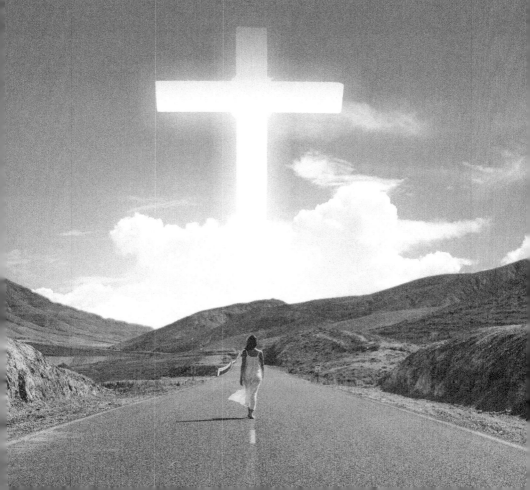

Chapter 4

NATURAL WAYS TO RESTORE HEALTH

How do you feel about your current medical treatment? If your health is getting worse, despite proper medical care, then it is wise to seek other natural therapies. God has designed our bodies with a powerful immune system and the ability to heal itself. However, for our body to function at its best, we must feed it properly and take good care of it. This includes proper nutrition, adequate sleep, exercise, and reducing stress.

It has been said that "Food is Medicine." What we eat has a direct effect on the type and severity of illness we face. Junk and processed foods have little or no nutritional value. Sugar can hinder and even paralyze our immune system, making it harder for our bodies to fight against diseases. Much of the food that is sold today has been genetically modified, contains harmful additives, and contains little or no nutrients that our body can use. This places tremendous stress on our bodies. Eating the right foods nourishes our bodies properly, gives us energy, and enables us to function the way God intended. When we eat the wrong foods, it forces our body to spend extra energy to metabolize and eliminate the toxins in those foods. Spending extra energy causes our body to become more tired and exhausted. Over a period of time, eating the wrong foods causes chronic inflammation in our bodies. This continual inflammatory response is the root cause of most of the chronic illnesses we face.

When Roger was diagnosed with colon cancer a few years ago, he had to make some big decisions. He had recently buried his mother who died from colon cancer. His mother had chemotherapy and had no improvement in fighting her cancer. His mother suffered intensely and had several complications from her chemotherapy. Roger was determined to seek healing from God in other ways. Roger decided to make a radical change to his diet. He ate a completely healthy diet, including juicing and supplements. Over a 3 to 6-month period, Roger felt better, regained strength, and his cancer decreased in size. By the end of one year, not only did all the cancer disappear, but Roger said he had no other health problems. He stated he was full of energy and felt the best he has ever felt in his entire life.

Each one of us has to take personal responsibility for our health. One of the best practical ways to start this journey into divine health is to develop a personal healing plan. Even minor changes can make a difference when they become a habit. As you implement some of these actions for your spirit, mind, and body, you will feel better.

The following are suggestions that you can include in your personal healing plan. Remember, even one or two actions in each area of spirit, mind, and body can result in improved health. When you make your plan, be sure to do what you enjoy and allow it to fit into your current life situation.

Ideas that you can use to improve your spiritual health.

1. Pray: talk to God about what you need and ask for His help
2. Read the Bible: find healing promises in the scriptures and speak them out loud over your life.
3. Fast: when done properly, fasting has great spiritual and physical benefits. It helps you draw closer to God and can help the body heal itself.

4. Listen to godly worship music: this is a great way to relieve stress and focus on God.

5. Serve someone else: as you help another person, the Lord blesses you.

Ideas that are good for a healthy mind.

1. Have an accountability group: one or two people who can help you, encourage you, and pray for you.

2. Schedule a fun activity: something you look forward to.

3. Read a good book: this can encourage you and can give you a fresh outlook or new ideas.

4. Find a good coach or counselor.

5. Get out of your usual space if possible: try to experience something new.

Ideas that support physical health.

1. Adequate sleep: our bodies heal during sleep.

2. Eat and drink as healthily as possible.

3. Exercise according to your ability: even a few minutes of regular walking is beneficial.

4. Avoid addictive drugs: these cause excess stress on the body.

5. Enjoy God's creation in nature: 10 to 15 minutes of exposure to sunlight can increase our vitamin D levels. Vitamin D is a powerful ally to our immune system's fight against disease.

After you develop a personal healing plan, it is time to turn to God and trust in Him. You need faith for your journey, which is discussed in the next chapter.

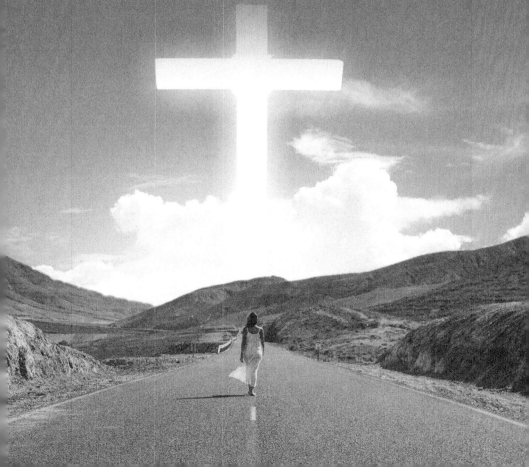

Chapter 5

FAITH OVER FEAR

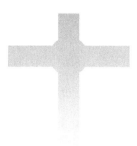

Have you received a negative medical report from your doctor? Does your sickness seem to get worse? In these situations, if we give into fear, it can paralyze us and hinder us from moving into divine health. The Bible tells us to walk by faith, not by sight. This means that we are to put our trust in God and His promises, and not in our natural circumstances.

Faith is a major key to experiencing divine health. Faith causes God to move on our behalf. People make mistakes that can interfere with their faith in God. When an individual rebels against God and refuses to repent of their sins, they hinder their faith. Things like unforgiveness, offense, idolatry, immorality, jealousy, and anger all can interfere with faith. God is not looking for perfection. He is simply looking for us to acknowledge our sins and confess them to Him. Sin breaks our relationship with God. God sent His Son, Jesus, to suffer and die on the cross for our sins. We deserve punishment for our sins, but Jesus paid the price for us so we can be free from the effects of sin. When we repent before God, He immediately forgives us and restores our relationship back to Himself.

Romans 10:9 reveals the simplicity of God's plan of salvation. This scripture verse tells us to confess with our mouth that Jesus is Lord and believe in our heart that God raised Him from the dead, and we will be saved. The first step to moving into divine health is to have a healthy spirit. So, if we want to experience divine health, we must start by receiving Jesus in our lives. Jesus renews our spirit when we receive Him, and His life flows into us. At the moment of salvation, our spirit becomes healthy, and we receive God's gift of eternal life. His presence dwells inside of us in a new and powerful way. God alone can renew our spirit.

If you have never received Jesus into your life, or you feel distant from Him, I encourage you to pray the following simple prayer out loud. Remember, it is not so much the words, but the sincerity of our heart as we say them.

Pray this prayer to receive Jesus or rededicate your life

to Him. "Lord Jesus, I know you are the Son of God. I acknowledge that I have sinned and made mistakes. You died on the cross to save me, and today I ask You to forgive me for my sins. I invite You to come into my life to be my Lord and Savior. Because You rose from the dead and are alive today, I know You are giving me an abundant life on earth. I also receive Your promise of eternal life in heaven. Thank You Jesus for saving me. Amen."

When you invite Jesus into your life, He will change you on the inside, and your life will never be the same. Jesus not only brings health and wholeness to your spirit, mind, and body, He also protects you from harm.

The following story illustrates how Jesus watches over us. I was driving my car and my eight-year-old son was in the front seat with me. We were driving to my older son's baseball game, and we stopped at an intersection. While waiting for the light to turn green, a large truck full of gravel smashed into the back of our car. The truck was going too fast and had some brake problems. My son and I never saw it coming. The impact of the truck was so great that it knocked our car forward about 50 feet. The trunk of our car was pushed into the second seat, every piece of glass in the car was shattered, and there was glass flying everywhere. A policeman, who was at the intersection, saw the entire accident. The policeman told me later that he thought whoever was in our car was probably dead. I can tell you that our God is greater! My son and I walked out of that car without a single scratch on us. The collision totaled the car, but we had no injuries.

I want you to know today that no matter what your illness or circumstances are, God is greater. There is nothing impossible for God, and it is His will for you to be healed. As you continue on this journey into divine health, you will know that God is always faithful. He said that He will never leave you or forsake you. Do not settle for poor health. When you believe God's promises for healing, it enables you to be confident of the future outcome. As you experience divine health, you will have a testimony of the goodness of God.

The healing process is frequently gradual. It often takes place in steps. It is important to recognize and celebrate success, no matter how insignificant it may seem. Your faith will grow step-by-step when you thank God for each improvement in your health. It is important to exercise your faith. That means you are to use the faith you have, even if it is only a small amount. As you put your faith into practice, it will grow little by little. Let me give you the following example.

If you are trying to build your muscle strength through lifting weights, you will start off with a small amount of weight. Over a period of time, as your muscles grow stronger, you will gradually increase the amount of weight you are lifting. If you continue with your weight training, you eventually get stronger and develop powerful muscle strength. The same principles are true with your faith. As you use your faith in your daily life and continue to exercise that faith, your faith will grow. As you persevere in using your faith, you will develop a strong faith. Just as it takes resistance from weights to build muscle strength, it also takes resistance from life's challenges to build the spiritual substance of faith.

God expects us to use our faith because faith is how we access the promises of God. Hebrews 6:12 reminds us that we inherit the promises of God through faith and patience. We must have faith in God and His Word and then persevere until we see God's promises manifested in our life. Exercising our faith is necessary for moving into divine health.

As your faith increases, you can ask God to heal one specific area in your life. This does not need to be the complete healing you are seeking. It can be simply one step in the process. It should be something that causes your faith to be stretched. Make it something that you can believe God for at this time. For example, if you have pain in multiple areas of your body, you can ask God to remove the pain in one area of your body. Then, as that area becomes pain free, you ask God to heal another area, etc. In this way, your faith will grow step-by-step. A faith that is increasing is ripe for miracles.

More about miracles can be found in the next chapter.

Chapter 6

DO YOU NEED A MIRACLE?

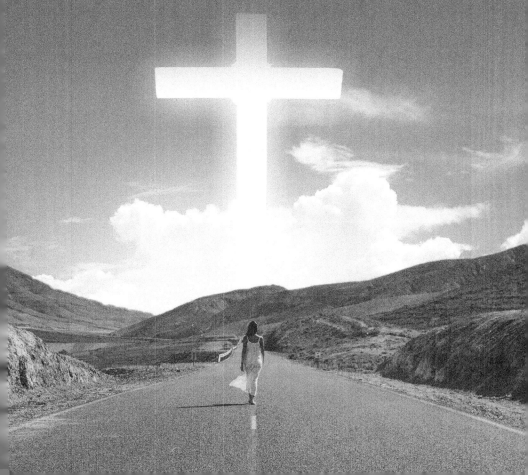

A re there no human answers for your illness or disease? I have good news for you. God is a miracle- working God. When it seems you have no place to turn for help, God is always there to do what no human can. Even now, God may be preparing you to receive a miracle. Our faith and trust need to be in God and His promises. Many times in the Bible, God tells us not to have fear or be anxious. God will always give you what you need at the right time if you turn to Him for help.

I have seen this happen many times in my career as a medical doctor. I was involved in several life-and-death situations where God intervened powerfully. As an anesthesiologist, I put people to sleep so they could have surgery. The vast majority of surgeries and anesthesia go very well, but some surgeries have complications. The following is a remarkable story of what God can do.

Suddenly, her heart stopped. What started as a routine day in the operating room turned into a day I will never forget. A middle-aged woman was asleep on the operating room table. The nurses were washing off her abdomen in order to sterilize it before surgery. Everything was going smoothly, and surgery had not started yet. Without warning, this woman's heart stopped. She was in complete cardiac arrest for no apparent reason. I called for help, and a team of people rushed into the operating room. I was maintaining the patient's breathing, and other people were giving CPR with chest compressions. The tension in the room was palpable. Over the next several minutes, the team was doing everything possible to save this woman's life. They gave multiple medications and electric shocks to restart her heart.

Multiple people witnessed that this woman was in cardiac arrest for 30 minutes. Even though CPR was being given, this was well beyond what would be compatible with life. After 30 minutes, the team was getting ready to stop all CPR. The surgeon had just left the operating room and was walking down the hall to talk to the patient's family.

Then the impossible happened. This woman's heart

started beating again. We all watched in utter amazement. This woman not only had a normal heart rhythm again, but also had a steady pulse and adequate blood pressure. A nurse ran to call the surgeon back to the operating room before he could talk to the family. Surgery was canceled, and this patient was transferred to the intensive care unit. Knowing that this woman was likely to have serious complications from her prolonged cardiac arrest, I was hoping and praying that God would intervene.

When I walked into this woman's room the next day, my jaw dropped. This woman was sitting up in bed, talking, and completely back to normal. My heart jumped inside of me as I thanked God for His goodness. When all our human efforts fall short, and we have nowhere else to turn, God will take over if we ask Him. No matter what illness you are struggling with or what difficulty you are facing, God is a miracle worker, and He has a miracle plan for you.

God desires to show His power in our daily lives. In Acts chapter 6, the Bible talks about Stephen, who worked a natural job as a waiter. God worked through him powerfully with miracles and healings. God often shows His power in what I would call a naturally supernatural way. This means an answer to a prayer or a physical healing often comes in a natural or unexpected way. If someone is not expecting God to heal them, or they are expecting God to heal them in a specific way, they can miss what God is doing for them.

I have found this to be true in many healing services that I have taken part in. I have seen people that were touched by God's healing power, and they did not even realize it. I have also seen people get disappointed when they do not receive an answer for their healing in the time frame they are expecting. God's timing differs from our human timing, but God's timing is always perfect. Isaiah 40:31 gives us valuable advice. This scripture tells us to renew our strength by waiting upon the Lord.

An important key to our healing is to trust God. We must have the expectation that He hears our prayers and will restore us. God works through medical professionals, natural remedies, and miraculous intervention. All ways of healing are available to God, and He is the ultimate source of healing. We must be patient during the healing process. God desires us to be healthy in our spirit, mind, and body. He may be bringing healing to our spirit and mind before our body is restored.

Do not give in to disappointment, doubt, or discouragement. Those are all negative emotions and thoughts that will hinder the healing process. Remember that Jesus suffered, died on the cross, and rose again to set us free from sin, sickness, and demonic spirits. The process of overcoming demonic spirits in an individual is called deliverance. There is a connection between healing and deliverance that I will discuss in the next chapter.

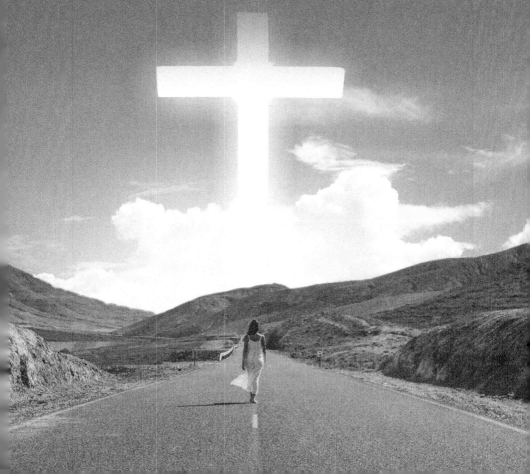

Chapter 7

DELIVERANCE IS AVAILABLE

D eliverance was a central part of the earthly ministry of Jesus. Deliverance involves setting people free from the negative or evil influences of demonic spirits. Demons are fallen angels who disobeyed God. The devil, otherwise known as Satan, oversees the demonic realm. Demons are constantly fighting against God and human beings because humans are created in the image of God. The good news is that when Jesus died on the cross and rose again, He totally defeated the devil so that people can now walk in freedom.

Jesus preached the Gospel of the Kingdom when He was on earth, and this message is still true today. The Gospel of the Kingdom is simply that what is in heaven is available to people on earth. In heaven, there is no sickness or disease, no hatred or anger, no evil spirits, and no unforgiveness. This means that those who receive the Kingdom message can experience the blessings of love, salvation, healing, and deliverance. Jesus not only preached the Kingdom message, but He also demonstrated the power of that Kingdom by healing the sick and casting out evil spirits. The same message and power of the Kingdom of God is available today to anyone who would like to receive it.

It is important to understand that there are different degrees of demonic influence seen in people. Demons can possess a person who is not a believer in Jesus. The devil cannot possess a Christian, but can oppress them. As previously explained, the spirit of the person who receives Jesus is immediately renewed at the moment of salvation. Therefore, evil spirits cannot control the spirit of a Christian. However, these demonic spirits can influence the mind and physical body of a Christian. This is what we call demonic influence or oppression on a believer in Jesus. For example, a Christian may have incorrect thinking about himself or about God. This person may believe certain lies that God does not love them, or they may not love themselves. This is an example of demonic influence on a person's mind, because they are not believing the truth.

When an individual receives Jesus as their Lord and Savior, their spirit is renewed. In addition, it is important for an individual to understand deliverance so they can walk in health in their mind and body.

There is a connection between healing and deliverance. Demons can cause sickness, but not all disease is caused by these evil spirits. Demonic influence was common in Jesus' day, and it is common today as well. Just as there is a wide range of severity in physical health problems, so there is a wide range of demonic influence. The more an individual lives in agreement with sin and lies, the more powerful the demonic influence on them will be.

Demons cannot simply inhabit, influence, or torment whomever they please. In order to gain access into a person's life, there must be an open door through which evil spirits oppress. An open door is simply an access point where evil spirits can influence a person. When we recognize how demons influence people, we can then shut those doors.

Some of the ways that people open the door to demonic influence in their lives are:

1. Embracing habitual sin
2. Experiencing the pain of abortion

3. Traumatic experiences, which include being sinned against. Even innocent victims of human trafficking, abuse, or abandonment can have evil spirits oppress them when the trauma against them is not healed.

4. Chronic unforgiveness, bitterness, or anger

5. Exposure to pornography

6. Involvement in ungodly sexual relationships

7. Involvement in the occult, false religions, or witch-craft is detrimental to your health and well-being.

8. Believing lies about ourselves or God.

Many people lack the knowledge that some things they are involved in are actually allowing the devil to attack them. Many of these doors can be shut through repentance, confessing our sins to the Lord, and forgiving those who have hurt us. A detailed discussion of how to experience freedom and healing through deliverance is beyond the scope of this book. If you need help in this area, I would encourage you to contact me personally through my website at www.divine-healingcoach.com/contact-me or find a good deliverance ministry.

I have worked with many people who have had health issues combined with demonic oppression. I worked with an older man who had chronic severe back pain for many years. After leading this man through a session on deliverance and closing doors he had opened, something incredible happened. Right after this man prayed with me, Jesus set him free from the demonic oppression, and instantly all his back pain was gone. There is power in the name of Jesus.

Because Jesus defeated the devil at the cross, you do not need to be afraid of demons. You have been given power and authority over evil spirits in the name of Jesus. Repentance must come first and then deliverance in order to experience the fullness of divine health.

Just like healings can be gradual or instantaneous, so deliverance can be instant or progressive. Deliverance can happen over a period of time because often the Lord wants to see an individual established in one area of freedom before moving on to the next area.

My hope is that the principles I have shared in this book can help you move into greater freedom and healing in your life. I am confident that by understanding and applying these biblical principles, you will experience healing in one or more areas of your life. My confidence does not rely on my own abilities, but it is based on Jesus and His promises in the Word of God. The greatest healing in your life comes when you experience the love of Jesus. In the next chapter, I will share the story of how Jesus visited me and changed my life. Jesus wants to change your life with His love.

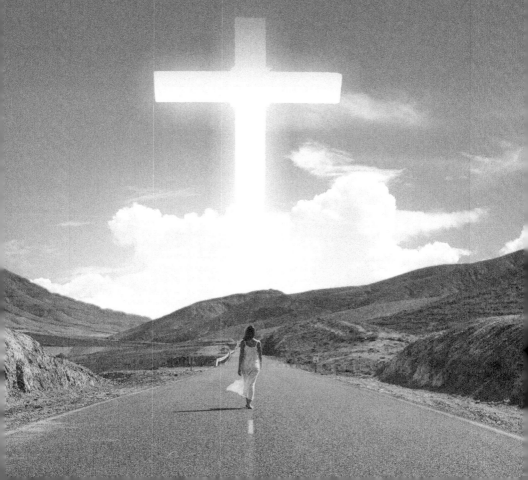

Chapter 8

JESUS LOVES YOU UNCONDITIONALLY

A night I will never forget! Jesus, the son of God, visited me. Before I share my story, I need to give you some biblical foundation for my experience with the Lord.

In 1 Kings 3:5-15, is the remarkable story of God appearing to Solomon in a dream. Solomon was the king of Israel. God asked him what he wanted, and Solomon asked God for wisdom. God was pleased with this request and gave Solomon wisdom, along with other blessings. A key point is that this was a dream, but when Solomon woke up, he had wisdom. When God the Father, Jesus, or the Holy Spirit visits someone, there is an impartation of the divine nature into that person.

Jesus appeared to me in a dream. During my sleep, I saw

Jesus in the prayer room of our ministry building. As soon as I saw Jesus in my dream, I cried out, "Jesus, Jesus," and He instantly appeared in front of me. I said, "I love You, I love You" and He hugged me, burying my face against His chest. In that embrace, I felt His unconditional love. Words are completely inadequate to describe what I experienced. I then woke up from the dream, and my body was visibly shaking for a minute or two. I also noticed that my belly was shaking. I asked the Lord to tell me what the shaking meant. Instantly I thought of the verses from John 7:37-38. In these Scriptures, Jesus says, "… If any man thirst, let him come unto Me and drink. He that believeth on Me, as the scripture hath said, out of his belly shall flow rivers of living water" (KJV).

The Lord blessed me so much through His visitation to me. His unconditional love has changed my life. It is His love for me that continually motivates me to love others. My passion is to connect you to this amazing love of Jesus and allow Him to heal your body, mind, and spirit. The love of Jesus will change you, heal you, and set you free. Jesus is offering you divine health. This includes victory over your illness and then remaining healthy. Are you ready to go on this journey with Jesus? Your life will never be the same.

ABOUT THE AUTHOR

After more than 30 years as a physician, Michael Peters, M.D. now travels the world releasing the message of divine health. He and his wife, Mary Jo, are known for their compassionate care for those who are sick, and they have helped thousands of people recover their health. God is working through Dr. Peters to bring miracles of healing to those in need.

Michael is the founder of Divine Healing Coaching which helps people struggling with sickness move into divine health. There are multiple resources available to help you restore your health. Free strategy sessions are designed to develop a personal plan for your healing. Training is available online on your own or with the encouragement of a coach.

For additional help or questions, contact Michael on Facebook @ Michael Peters or on his website:

www.divinehealingcoach.com/coaching
www.divinehealingcoach.com/online-training